THE DHEA BIOLOGICAL SYSTEM

Understanding The Function Of Dhea In Biological System, Equilibrium Of Hormones, Types, Benefits & Side Effects, Safety Measures & More

Nuel Nenji

1

Table of Contents

Introductory

Both the adrenal glands, which are situated on top of each kidney, are responsible for the production of the steroid hormone known as dehydroepiandrosterone (DHEA).

It has a role in the creation of other hormones, such as testosterone and estrogen, by acting as a precursor. As people get older, their levels of DHEA tend to steadily decrease after reaching their peak in early adulthood.

Over the years, DHEA has garnered attention in a variety of fields, including the control of mood, the process of aging, and overall health and wellness. On the other hand, some individuals take DHEA supplements in an effort to improve their athletic performance or to address concerns that are associated with aging.

On the other hand, the scientific evidence that supports the usefulness and safety of DHEA supplementation is not absolutely conclusive, and the effects that occur over a longer period of time are not completely known.

It is essential to keep in mind that DHEA is regarded as a prohibited substance in certain countries;

hence, the inclusion of this ingredient in dietary supplements must to be addressed with caution. When contemplating the use of any hormonal supplement, it is recommended to first consult with a qualified medical practitioner in order to evaluate the potential risks and benefits of the supplement based on the specific health requirements and conditions of the individual.

CHAPTER ONE
DHEA Levels In The Human Body

The adrenal glands, which are located on top of each kidney, are the primary organs responsible for the production of the steroid hormone known as dehydroepiandrosterone (DHEA).

It is also synthesized in the brain and the gonads, which are the reproductive organs that include the ovaries and the testicles. In addition to its function as a precursor to the sex hormones testosterone and estrogen,

DHEA is also involved in a number of other physiological processes that occur within the human body. The following is a list of important characteristics of DHEA in the body:

- DHEA is a precursor to the hormones that are associated with sexuality. It is transformed into other hormones, such as testosterone and estrogen. The regulation of the menstrual cycle, the maintenance of bone density, and the development of secondary sexual traits are all influenced by these sex hormones, which play important roles in all three instances.

- The levels of DHEA in the body are known to reach their highest point throughout the early years of adulthood, and then these levels steadily decrease as one gets older. DHEA levels can be much lower by the time individuals reach their 70s and 80s when compared to early stages of life than they were in earlier stages.

- DHEA is secreted by the adrenal glands in response to stimulation by adrenocorticotropic hormone (ACTH), which helps the adrenal glands perform their function. The pituitary gland is responsible for the production of ACTH, which is a component of the body's stress response system.

- Cognitive Function: Several research have investigated the possible connections that exist between DHEA levels and performance in cognitive tasks. It is important to note that the connection between DHEA and cognitive health is a complicated one that is not completely understood.

- With regard to immunological function, it is believed that DHEA plays a part in the regulation of the immune system; however, the mechanisms involved are not completely understood.

- Anti-Aging Hypothesis: Some people have investigated the possibility that taking DHEA supplements could have anti-aging effects or a positive impact on overall well-being. On the other hand, the scientific evidence that can be used to support these statements is equivocal, and additional research is required to fully comprehend the potential advantages and disadvantages.

- Health disorders: Certain health disorders, such as adrenal insufficiency or adrenal tumors, have the potential to affect the levels of DHEA in the body. Under the guidance of a medical professional, DHEA supplementation may be administered in some circumstances in order to address particular health concerns.

While it is true that DHEA can be purchased as a supplement, it is essential to emphasize that its utilization need to be addressed with caution, particularly in the absence of appropriate medical management.

It is possible for taking hormone supplements to have a variety of complex impacts on the body, and the responses of different people can vary. When contemplating the use of DHEA supplements, it is recommended to first discuss the matter with a qualified medical practitioner.

Functions Of DHEA In Biological Systems

Within the human body, dehydroepiandrosterone, often known as DHEA, is responsible for a number of crucial biological processes. Key roles include the following:

- DHEA is a precursor to the creation of sex hormones such as testosterone and estrogen. It contributes to the development of these hormones by acting as a precursor. These hormones are necessary for the creation of secondary sexual characteristics, the maintenance of reproductive health, and the maintenance of hormonal equilibrium in general.

- Effects on Aging and Anti-Aging: DHEA levels typically reach their highest point in early adulthood and then begin to decrease as one gets older. The possibility that preserving or augmenting DHEA levels could have anti-aging effects has been investigated by a number of studies.

- On the other hand, the connection between DHEA and the aging process is a complicated one, and the scientific evidence that supports claims of anti-aging is not conclusive.

- In the context of immune system regulation, it is believed that DHEA plays a part in the modulation of the immune system. The possibility that DHEA may have immunomodulatory effects, which would mean that it would influence the activity of immune cells, has been proposed. On the other hand, thorough comprehension of the specific mechanisms is lacking.

- Within the realm of cognitive function, there is a certain amount of curiosity regarding the possible impact that DHEA could play. Although there have been some studies that have investigated the connections between DHEA levels and various elements of cognitive function, the relationship between the two is not well-established, and additional study is required to define the impact that DHEA has on cognitive health.

- As a result of the stimulation provided by adrenocorticotropic hormone (ACTH), the adrenal glands secrete DHEA in response to the stress that they experience. It is a component of the stress response system in the body and plays a role in the adaptation of the body to the many stressors that it encounters.

- Health of the Bones: Sex hormones, particularly those that are generated from DHEA, have a role in the maintenance of bone density over time. It is therefore possible that DHEA has an indirect influence on bone health.

- On the subject of mood regulation, a number of research have been conducted to investigate the possible effects of DHEA on mental health and well-being. On the other hand, the evidence is contradictory, and additional research is required to establish a definitive connection between DHEA levels and the capability to regulate mood.

While it is true that DHEA can be purchased as a supplement, it is essential to emphasize that its utilization need to be addressed with proper caution. It is possible for individuals to experience different results when taking DHEA supplements, and taking excessive amounts of DHEA may have negative consequences.

In addition, the efficacy and safety of DHEA supplementation over the long term are not well recognized. When contemplating the use of DHEA supplements, it is recommended to get the advice of a qualified medical practitioner in order to ascertain whether or not they are suitable for the individual's current state of health and requirements.

CHAPTER TWO
DHEA And The Equilibrium Of Hormones

Dehydroepiandrosterone, often known as DHEA, is a hormone that is a precursor to the sex hormones testosterone and estrogen. Additionally, it plays a function in maintaining the body's hormonal equilibrium.

The maintenance of hormonal equilibrium is essential for a variety of physiological activities, including the regulation of mood, reproductive health, and overall general well-being.

According to the following, DHEA helps maintain hormonal equilibrium:

- Production of Testosterone and Estrogen: The body's enzymatic systems are responsible for the conversion of DHEA into both testosterone and estrogen. In contrast to estrogen, which plays a significant role in the reproductive health of women, testosterone is an essential male sex hormone. Both of these hormones, in their own unique ways, provide a contribution to the preservation of hormonal equilibrium.

- Health of the Reproductive System It is vital for both men and women to have healthy levels of sex hormones in order to maintain reproductive health. Estrogen is essential for the menstrual cycle and fertility in females, whereas testosterone is essential for the creation of sperm and the overall reproductive function in males.

- Support for Menopause: When it comes to women,

DHEA has been investigated as a possible supplement that could help maintain hormonal equilibrium during menopause.

It is possible that DHEA will help to maintain a more balanced hormonal profile for women when estrogen levels continue to decrease. On the other hand, the use of DHEA during menopause is a subject of continuing research, and individual reactions may result in different outcomes.

- Function of the Adrenal System: The adrenal glands

are responsible for the production of DHEA, in addition to other hormones that are involved in the body's response to stress. In order to keep the hormonal balance in the body in check and to react effectively to stressors, it is necessary that the adrenal glands work properly.

- Balance between androgens and estrogens: It is essential for both men and women to ensure that they have a healthy equilibrium between androgens (such as testosterone) and estrogens in order to protect their overall health. By acting as a precursor to both types of hormones, DHEA makes a contribution to maintaining this equilibrium.

- When it comes to maintaining hormonal equilibrium, it is essential to keep in mind that although DHEA can be purchased as a supplement, its utilization should be addressed with caution. Taking hormone supplements can have a wide range of consequences since the hormonal systems in the body are so intricately interconnected. In addition, the responses of individuals to DHEA supplementation can vary, and there is a possibility that excessive quantities of sex hormones could have negative consequences.

It is recommended that you get the advice of a qualified medical expert before contemplating the use of DHEA supplements or any other hormonal intervention whatsoever. Their ability to evaluate your individual health situation, describe the potential dangers and benefits, and offer recommendations regarding whether or not such supplementation is suitable for your particular requirements is a significant advantage. While maintaining hormonal equilibrium is a delicate and highly individualized element of health, it is essential to seek the help of a specialist in order to successfully navigate these complexities.

DHEA's Positive Effects On Health

Research has been conducted on dehydroepiandrosterone (DHEA) in order to investigate the possible positive effects it may have on one's health. It is essential to keep in mind that although there are particular studies that point to good impacts, the evidence is frequently contradictory, and additional study is required to arrive at conclusive findings. Some of the areas in which DHEA has been investigated for its possible positive effects on health are as follows:

- DHEA levels have a tendency to decrease with age, which led to the theory that taking a supplement containing DHEA could potentially have anti-aging effects. There have been a few studies that have showed that using DHEA supplements may improve the health of the skin, boost cognitive performance, and lower the chance of developing age-related disorders. However, additional research is required to be sure that these possible benefits are accurate.

- Health of the Bones: Sex hormones, particularly those that are generated from DHEA, have a role in the maintenance of bone density over time. A number of research have investigated the connection between DHEA levels and bone health, and the findings of these studies suggest that taking DHEA supplements may have a beneficial effect, particularly in women who have gone through menopause.

- On the other hand, additional research is required to determine whether or not DHEA is both effective and safe for optimizing bone health.

- Mood and Mental Health: There is some research that suggests that DHEA may have beneficial impacts on both the feelings of happiness and the mental health of individuals. Research has been conducted on its effects on mental health issues such as anxiety and depression, and some of the findings suggest that it may have potential advantages.

- Health of the Metabolic System: DHEA has been examined for its possible involvement in enhancing insulin sensitivity and nutritional health of the metabolic system. There are some studies that have suggested that taking DHEA supplements might have a good impact on glucose metabolism; however, the evidence is not consistent, and there is a need for additional research.

- There have been a few research that have investigated the potential impact that DHEA may have on libido and sexual function. DHEA is involved in the generation of sex hormones, and these studies have studied its potential impact. On the other hand, the results are contradictory, and the consequences may be different for different people.

- Although there is some exciting research on the possible health advantages of DHEA, it is essential to note that the evidence is not solid or consistent across all trials. This is something that has to be emphasized.

Additionally, there is the potential for adverse effects and interactions with drugs when taking DHEA supplements. Therefore, it is recommended to get the advice of a qualified medical practitioner before contemplating the use of DHEA supplements for any particular health purpose.

It is possible for them to offer individualized guidance that is based on the current state of an individual's health and to assist in weighing the potential benefits and hazards of DHEA supplementation.

CHAPTER THREE
Effects And Dangers That Could Be Involved

Even though dehydroepiandrosterone (DHEA) has been investigated for the possibility of having positive impacts on health, it is essential to be aware of the potential hazards and adverse consequences that are linked with its utilization. It is important to keep in mind that different people will have different answers, and the material that follows is intended to provide a basic overview:

- An imbalance in hormone levels may occur as a result of

treatment with DHEA, which is a precursor to sex hormones. This imbalance may be caused by testosterone and estrogen levels. Alterations in mood, libido, and reproductive health are just some of the possibilities that might arise as a result of this imbalance.

- Acne and Oily Skin: High amounts of DHEA has been linked to increased oil production in the skin, which may be a contributing factor in the development of acne and oily skin.

- There is a possibility that some people will experience hair loss as a consequence of taking DHEA supplements, particularly if the supplement causes an increase in the levels of androgen in their bodies.

- Insomnia and Sleep Disturbances: Because DHEA can have stimulating effects, it is possible that some people will have trouble sleeping or experiencing insomnia when they take DHEA supplements, particularly if they are taken later in the day.

- Concerns have been raised regarding the potential effect that DHEA supplementation may have on lipid metabolism and the health of the cardiovascular system. There are several research that point to the possibility of effects on cholesterol levels, but the evidence is not consistent and contradictory.

- It is possible that taking DHEA supplements for an extended period of time could have an effect on the function of the liver. It is essential for those who have illnesses that affect the liver or who are taking medications that have an effect on the liver to take caution.

- Hormone-Sensitive Conditions: Because DHEA has the ability to affect hormone levels, those who have hormone-sensitive conditions, such as some forms of cancers (for example, breast and prostate cancer), should avoid using DHEA supplements without the guidance of a medical professional.

- Interactions with drugs: Numerous drugs, such as hormone treatments, antidepressants, and corticosteroids, have the potential to interact with DHEA supplements. Before using DHEA, it is essential to discuss the medicine with a qualified medical expert, particularly if you are also taking other prescriptions.

- Some populations, such as women who are pregnant or lactating, should avoid taking DHEA supplements because they are not advised for everyone. DHEA supplements are not recommended for everyone. Individuals who have a history of hormone-related malignancies, cardiac disorders, or liver difficulties should exercise caution and seek the opinion of a medical professional beforehand.

Additionally, it is essential to emphasize that the use of DHEA supplements should be done so under the supervision of a qualified medical practitioner. In the absence of adequate supervision, self-prescribing DHEA might result in unforeseen consequences and increase the likelihood of adverse health effects. If you are thinking about taking DHEA supplements for a particular health issue, you should talk to your healthcare practitioner about the potential benefits, risks, and dosages that are appropriate for you depending on your current state of health.

In the event that you choose to take DHEA supplements, it is imperative that you undergo consistent monitoring and follow-up with a qualified medical practitioner.

Different Kinds Of DHEA Supplements

It is possible for individuals to select different types of dehydroepiandrosterone (DHEA) supplements according on their preferences and requirements. These supplements are available in a variety of formats. Notable examples of DHEA supplements include the following:

- Among the several forms of DHEA supplements, the most popular and commonly available form is that of DHEA pills or capsules. Individuals often take them with water, and they are available in the form of capsules or pills that are taken orally. A daily supplement habit can easily be incorporated into this format because it is practical and easy to use.

- The topical forms of DHEA, such as creams and gels, are preferred by some individuals to the topical forms of DHEA. After being applied to the skin, these formulations allow the DHEA to be absorbed into the bloodstream through the skin. For individuals who have difficulties swallowing tablets or who would rather avoid taking oral supplements, topical applications may offer an alternative means of administration.

- DHEA that is administered sublingually: Sublingual supplements are intended to be dissolved completely under the tongue. For this reason, it is possible for the DHEA to be absorbed directly into the bloodstream through the mucous membranes that are found in the mouth. It is possible that those who wish to avoid the digestive system and obtain rapid absorption will prefer sublingual formulations of the medication.

- There are liquid formulations of DHEA that can be found in the form of drops. DHEA drops are also available in liquid form. It is possible for users to measure the dosage that they want and then combine it with water or another beverage.

People who have trouble swallowing pills or who like the flexibility of being able to change their dosage may find that liquid formulations are something that they can use.

- Pellets or Implants of DHEA: DHEA may be provided in the form of pellets or implants that are put beneath the skin in some instances. DHEA is released into the bloodstream in a gradual manner by these pellets over a prolonged length of time. There are fewer instances of this approach being used, and it might require a medical treatment to insert.

Before beginning a regimen, persons who are contemplating the use of

DHEA supplements should, regardless of the form, check with a healthcare expert. This is an essential point to keep in mind. It is possible for DHEA supplements to have varied rates of absorption, as well as the potential to mix with drugs or have different effects on various people.

Furthermore, the ideal dosage and type of DHEA can be determined by a variety of criteria, including the individual's age, gender, current state of health, and the particular health objectives that they wish to achieve.

It is essential to select a reliable brand and adhere to the dosages that are prescribed, just as it is with any other supplement. In order to guarantee that the usage of DHEA supplements is both safe and effective, it is important to maintain regular monitoring and discussion with a healthcare expert.

CHAPTER FOUR
Considerations & Safety Measures To Take

When contemplating the utilization of DHEA supplements, it is essential to take into account a number of factors and dangers associated with the product. To keep in mind, the following are some important points:

- Consultation with a Healthcare practitioner It is essential to consult with a healthcare practitioner prior to beginning any kind of supplementation that contains DHEA. The significance of this cannot be overstated due to the fact that DHEA has the ability to affect hormone levels, and the usage of this substance may have varying impacts on various people depending on characteristics such as age, gender, and overall health.

- An Individualized Approach: The administration of DHEA supplements have to be done on an individual basis. It is possible for dosages to change depending on the particular health objectives of the individual, and the appropriate dosage might be affected by characteristics such as age, gender, and preexisting health issues.

- Monitoring Hormone Levels It is recommended that individuals who are taking DHEA supplements engage in regular monitoring of their hormone levels. This has the potential to assist in maintaining hormone levels within a healthy range and can provide information that can be used to inform any necessary alterations to the supplementing approach.

- Possible Interactions with drugs: DHEA supplements have the potential to interact with a wide range of drugs, such as hormone treatments, antidepressants, and corticosteroids. You should be sure to inform your healthcare practitioner about all of the medications and supplements that you are currently taking so that they can evaluate the possibility of any interactions.

- Hormone-Sensitive Conditions: Individuals who have hormone-sensitive conditions, such as some forms of cancers (for example, breast and prostate cancer), should avoid taking DHEA supplements without the guidance of a medical professional. As a result of its ability to affect hormone levels, the use of DHEA in such circumstances may make certain conditions even worse.

- It is possible that taking DHEA supplements for an extended period of time could have an effect on the function of the liver. It is important for those who already have liver issues or who are taking medications that have an effect on the liver to exercise caution and seek the advice of a qualified medical expert.

- Adverse Effects: Although DHEA is generally believed to be safe when used appropriately, it is possible for it to have adverse effects such as acne, greasy skin, hair loss, and changes in mood. Immediately seeking the advice of a healthcare expert is essential in the event that any unfavorable consequences are observed.

- It is not recommended that women who are pregnant or breastfeeding take DHEA supplements because of the potential impact that they could have on their hormone levels. Women who are pregnant should steer clear of DHEA unless they have received explicit instructions from a medical professional.

- Supplemental Quality It is important to select DHEA supplements from reliable suppliers in order to guarantee the quality of the product and the correctness of the dosages. When shopping for dietary supplements, it is recommended to choose products from well-known brands that adhere to excellent manufacturing operations.

It is important to keep in mind that DHEA is a hormone, and that taking hormone supplements can have a wide range of impacts on the body. In order to ensure the highest level of safety, it is essential to approach the use of DHEA with caution, under the supervision of a qualified medical practitioner, and to emphasize safety by monitoring for potential adverse effects and interactions. People who are contemplating or already utilizing DHEA supplements should make it a priority to follow up with their healthcare professional on a regular basis.

Production Of DHEA With The Help Of Nutritional Support

The adrenal glands are responsible for the synthesis of a hormone known as dehydroepiandrosterone (DHEA). The production of this hormone is affected by a number of factors, one of which is nutrition. It is true that there is no diet that specifically promotes DHEA production; nevertheless, maintaining general health by consuming a diet that is both well-balanced and abundant in nutrients can help the body's natural hormone production. The following are some dietary considerations that may assist the generation of DHEA as well as the overall health of the endocrine system:

- Foods High in Protein: Consuming an adequate amount of protein is necessary for the creation of hormones to occur, including DHEA. Lean protein can be obtained from a variety of sources, including poultry, fish, lean meats, eggs, dairy products, legumes, and plant-based proteins. Include these sources in your diet.

- Healthy Fats: Make sure that your diet contains a variety of types of healthy fats, such as monounsaturated fats and omega-3 fatty acids. These fats play a crucial role in the production of hormones. Olive oil, flaxseeds, chia seeds, walnuts, avocados, and fatty fish (salmon and mackerel) are some examples of foods that should be considered.

- Zinc is a mineral that is involved in the manufacture of a number of hormones, including DHEA. Foods that are rich in zinc are found in this category. Items such as oysters, red meat, poultry, dairy products, nuts, and seeds are examples of foods that are high in zinc.

- Vitamin C: Vitamin C is an antioxidant that helps the adrenal glands function properly and can also assist in the process of converting DHEA into other hormones. Make sure that your diet contains foods like bell peppers, broccoli, kiwi, citrus fruits, and berries.

- Vitamins B: vitamins B, in particular B5 (pantothenic acid) and B6 (pyridoxine), play a role in the function of the adrenal glands and the generation of hormones. There are a variety of foods that are rich in B vitamins, including whole grains, meat, chicken, fish, nuts, seeds, and leafy green vegetables.

- Consuming foods that are high in magnesium is important because magnesium has a role in the regulation of adrenal hormones. Be sure to incorporate foods that are high in magnesium into your diet, such as legumes, nuts, seeds, and whole grains, as well as leafy green vegetables.

- Adaptogenic Herbs: It is believed that certain herbs possess adaptogenic characteristics, which assist the body in adjusting to stress and may also boost adrenal function. As an illustration, holy basil, rhodiola, and ashwagandha are all examples.

In traditional medicine, these herbs are frequently utilized; nevertheless, prior to utilizing them as dietary supplements, it is essential to seek the advice of a qualified medical practitioner.

- One of the most important aspects of general health, including the functioning of the adrenal glands, is maintaining an adequate level of hydration. Throughout the course of the day, you should be sure to consume a sufficient amount of water.

Although maintaining a balanced diet is an essential component of not just overall well-being but also hormonal health, it is essential to keep in mind that individual reactions can differ.

In addition, it is recommended that you get the advice of a trained dietitian or a healthcare expert if you are contemplating making large alterations to your diet or if you have specific health issues. They are able to provide individualized assistance that is tailored to your specific health status and requirements.

CHAPTER FIVE
What Effect Does Physical Activity Have On DHEA Levels?

The practice of regular exercise has the potential to have a beneficial effect on one's general health, including the potential to influence hormone levels.

Despite the fact that the connection between physical activity and levels of dehydroepiandrosterone (DHEA) is a complicated one that can vary from person to person, there is some evidence to suggest that some types of physical activity may have an effect on the synthesis of DHEA.

Take into consideration the following points:

- Aerobic Exercise: It has been found that engaging in aerobic exercise on a regular basis, through activities such as running, cycling, or brisk walking, has been connected with good impacts on DHEA levels.

  There is evidence that aerobic exercise is beneficial to cardiovascular health and may also contribute to the maintenance of hormonal equilibrium.

- Strength exercise: There is evidence from a number of studies that suggests that resistance exercise, generally known as weightlifting, may also have a beneficial effect on DHEA levels.

  A number of hormones, including DHEA, may be influenced by resistance training, which is associated with increased muscle mass and strength. Resistance training may also impact body composition.

- Intensity and Duration: Both the intensity of the exercise and the length of time it is performed may have an effect on the hormonal response. Both moderate-intensity and high-intensity exercise have been investigated, and some studies have suggested that higher intensity may have a more significant influence on DHEA levels than moderate-intensity exercise.

- Alterations that are Associated with Age: The levels of DHEA naturally decrease with age, and the effects of exercise on DHEA may vary depending on whether the individual is younger or older. It has been shown in a few studies that physical activity may aid to prevent the fall in DHEA levels that is associated with aging.

- Intense or prolonged exercise can be a source of physical stress on the body, and cortisol might be increased as a result of this stress. In contrast to acute stress, which can stimulate the production of DHEA, chronic stress, which can include overtraining, can lead to higher cortisol levels, which can have an effect on DHEA values. To prevent the body from experiencing an excessive amount of stress, it is essential to keep up a well-balanced workout regimen.

- Variability at the Individual Level: Different people can have different reactions to physical activity. Whether or not exercise has an effect on DHEA levels is contingent upon a number of factors, including genetics, general health, and individual variances in the way hormones are regulated.

- The fact that exercise can be helpful for overall health and may have positive impacts on hormone levels is something that should be taken into consideration.

  However, it is crucial to highlight that excessive or severe activity without proper recuperation can lead to bad health results. The idea is to include both aerobic and resistance training in your workout program in order to achieve a well-rounded fitness routine that strikes a balance.

As is always the case, judgments about exercise should be guided by individual health factors. In the event that you are experiencing certain health issues or are contemplating making significant modifications to your workout program, it is highly recommended that you seek the advice of a healthcare professional or a fitness specialist.

They are able to offer coaching that is individualized to your specific requirements and assist in ensuring that your approach to exercise is both safe and successful.

Controlling Stress And Taking DHEA

The strategies that are used to manage stress can have a substantial impact on a variety of elements of health, including fluctuations in hormone levels.

The hormone known as dehydroepiandrosterone (DHEA), which is produced by the adrenal glands, is affected by one's level of stress as well as the body's reaction to stresses. The following are some of the ways in which stress management may be related to levels of DHEA.

- Both cortisol and DHEA are produced by the adrenal glands in reaction to stress. This might be considered a balance between the two hormones.

Cortisol levels can be elevated as a result of chronic or persistent stress, which can then have an effect on DHEA levels. There are two hormones that are frequently referred to as "counter-regulatory" hormones: cortisol and DHEA. It is essential for general hormonal health to maintain a balance between these two hormones.

- Adaptogenic Herbs: It is believed that certain herbs, which are referred to as adaptogens, can assist the body in adapting to stress and possess the potential to impact the equilibrium of cortisol and DHEA.

Research has been conducted to investigate the potential effects that adaptogens such as ashwagandha, rhodiola, and holy basil may have on the functioning of the stress response system.

- Mind-Body Practices: Studies have shown that practices like yoga, meditation, and deep breathing exercises are connected with lower levels of stress and may have a good affect on DHEA levels.

Several studies have demonstrated that these practices have the ability to alter the activity of the hypothalamic-pituitary-adrenal (HPA) axis, which is an essential component of the body's reaction to emotional stress.

- Frequent Physical Activity: Engaging in regular physical activity can serve as a method of stress management and may also contribute to the maintenance of hormonal equilibrium.

  Researchers have found that exercise has a good impact on DHEA levels, particularly when it is incorporated into a comprehensive routine that is performed at a moderate intensity.

- Getting Enough Sleep: Prolonged exposure to stress can have a detrimental effect on one's ability to sleep, and not getting enough sleep can lead to imbalances in cortisol and DHEA levels. It is possible that one of the most significant aspects of stress management is making excellent sleep hygiene a priority and getting appropriate amounts of sleep.

- A diet that is both well-balanced and rich in nutrients can be beneficial to one's general health and can assist the body in managing stress. Consuming foods that are rich in nutrients provide the essential components that are required for the manufacture of hormones, including DHEA.

- There is a correlation between having strong social ties and having social support, which is responsible for better stress management. It is possible to have a beneficial influence on one's total well-being, including her hormonal health, by participating in constructive social interactions and having a support system.

The fact that different people have different reactions to stress and different ways of dealing with it is something that must be acknowledged. In spite of the fact that stress management may have a beneficial impact on DHEA levels for certain individuals, other individuals may require a combination of strategies that are specifically suited to their exceptional circumstances.

If stress is a serious worry for you, and especially if you are contemplating specific therapies such as adaptogenic herbs or supplements, it is recommended that you seek the advice of a healthcare practitioner. They are able to provide individualized guidance and assistance in determining the most suitable interventions for stress management and the maintenance of hormonal equilibrium, taking into account the specific requirements of your health.

Summary

To summarize, dehydroepiandrosterone, often known as DHEA, is a steroid hormone that is produced by the adrenal glands. It plays a role as a precursor to sex hormones such as testosterone and estrogen.

As a result of its many functions within the body, it has an impact on a variety of elements, including reproductive health, immunological function, mood management, and overall healthy functioning.

It is important to note that the connection between DHEA and these processes is a complicated one, and the scientific understanding of the effects of DHEA is still in the process of developing.

Research has been conducted to investigate the possible health benefits of DHEA supplementation. These potential benefits include anti-aging effects, support for cognitive function, and improvements in mood and other aspects of well-being. There is a lack of consistency in the evidence, and the long-term consequences of DHEA supplementation are not completely understood, despite the fact that certain studies have suggested advantageous outcomes.

Furthermore, DHEA supplements have the potential to cause adverse effects and interact with other medications, highlighting the significance of exercising caution and seeking the advice of a qualified practitioner.

Exercising, managing stress, maintaining a healthy diet, and getting enough sleep are all factors that might have an effect on DHEA levels and contribute to the overall hormonal balance.

When it comes to maintaining a healthy lifestyle, crucial components include engaging in regular physical activity, adopting stress management strategies, maintaining a balanced diet, and prioritizing appropriate sleep. These are all things that have the potential to favorably improve both DHEA and overall well-being.

The fact that different people have different reactions to DHEA and lifestyle modifications highlights the significance of taking a highly individualized strategy. It is imperative to get the advice of a qualified medical practitioner before making any significant adjustments to one's living patterns or before contemplating the use of DHEA supplements.

They are able to evaluate the current state of an individual's health, offer advice on the possible risks and benefits, and assist in tailoring actions to meet particular requirements.

In order to successfully navigate the complexity of hormones and health, it is essential to take a cautious and well-informed approach. For the purpose of ensuring optimal health and well-being, it is essential to maintain consistent communication with medical professionals, to perform continuous monitoring, and to make adjustments depending on feedback received from individuals.

THE END

Manufactured by Amazon.ca
Acheson, AB